YOUR *Body* AS THE *Creation* of CONSCIOUSNESS

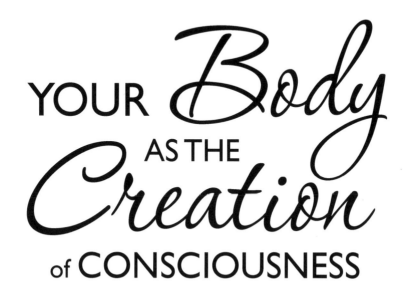

YOUR *Body* AS THE *Creation* of CONSCIOUSNESS

PATTY ALFONSO

SECRET BONUSES JUST FOR YOU!

As a special thank you for buying my book, I'd like to invite you to be a part of my *Secret Bonuses Membership* page.

To access the site for free go to:

YourBodyIsConsciousneness.com/secretbonuses

and enter your email address.

I've created a place with additional resources, inspirational videos and quotes, some samples of what Pole Dancing For Consciousness™ looks like, meditations and receiving exercises and much more!

When you join my list you'll also receive articles, video content and special invitations to all of my upcoming webinars, classes and exclusive live events.

These resources will guide you in having more joy, sensation, pleasure and fun in your life.

What if the purpose of life is to have fun?!

Enjoy these gifts. Thank you again for purchasing my book!

I hope to see you, someday, around the globe!

Dedication

To my family, for creating the space for me to thrive, grow and choose to be all of me. I am so grateful for you!

To all of my friends, from every stage of my life, thank you for being there. Thank you for all the laughs, the fun and having my back!

To Irvin, Linda, Malka, Chava, Ari and Yaakov, thank you for saving my life. I adore you infinitely!

To Gary and Dain, thank you for never quitting, never giving up and never stopping.

Acknowledgement

I would like to acknowledge the tools of Access Consciousness®.

I have been seeking since 2007.

In all of my years studying and learning different tools and techniques for healing, these tools have been the most fun and the easiest to use!

You can apply the tools of Access Consciousness® to anything you are looking to change about your life.

A miraculous body of work, the tools include verbal processes as well as over 60 body processes to include your body on your journey towards consciousness.

For more information about the tools, go to:

www.AccessConsciousness.com
www.DrDainHeer.com
www.GaryMDouglas.com

Awaken (v)

To spring into being, arise, originate. To wake up. To rouse from sleep. To stir up, rouse to activity.

Embody (v)

In reference to a spirit invested with a physical form. To give a bodily form to; incarnate. To represent in a clear and obvious way.

Unleash (v)

Release from a leash or restraint. To become unrestrained. To suddenly release a force that cannot be controlled.

9

Your body IS consciousness.

You are consciousness embodied.

We have seen ourselves as separate from our bodies for millennia.

As we move forward and open up to embodied consciousness, we can move into total communion with our bodies.

There is the consciousness of your Body and there is the consciousness of you the Being.

What if there was no separation between the two?

You chose your body to create with in this lifetime...

*Are you creating with your body
or against your body?*

*What if you invited the consciousness of your
body to contribute to your life and living?*

Contents

Prologue

I grew up in an upper-middle class Latin home in Puerto Rico. My father was Cuban and my mother was Puerto Rican. To everyone around us we were the perfect family. My sister and I did not lack anything financially.

We were blessed to have a very hard-working father who provided all of the comforts that this reality had to offer.

I attended an all girls private school from Kindergarten through 12th grade. I don't recall much from my early years (more on this later).

The first time I really perceived the energy of my childhood was during my years at an energy healing school in Los Angeles, CA. We were assigned an exercise. The exercise was to perceive our childhood and describe what we sensed energetically. As I sat with a baby picture in my hand and perceived the past, I recalled a pervasive sense of danger, fear and anger.

Sitting outside on the grass, under the sunlight, surrounded by glorious trees, all I could perceive was darkness.

I wasn't exactly surprised at this perception. I had spent my teenage years through my thirties under the influence of drugs and alcohol in order to numb the awareness' of my childhood.

What did surprise me was the awareness that the energy I was perceiving was not mine. I was acutely aware that this was the way my Mom and Dad had chosen to create their lives.

Later in life I became aware I had chosen them so I could thrive beyond them. The suppressed anger, fear and rage that I had grown up with was so obvious that suddenly everything seemed to make sense.

At the time of this recollection, I did not have the tools of Access Consciousness®. These glorious tools came to me 5 years later.

I had been at the energy healing school for 4 years, taken every class twice, certified three times over, begun my private healing business and I was BORED!

I knew there had to be more to this life than re-telling the sad story of the black sheep in the family no one had ever listened to. Plus, the healing process was sloooooowwwwww.....

And so here I am, now, with you.

I'd like to share with you my adventure in discovering the joy of living, the joy of having a body and the ways in which dancing contributed to the creation of the life I always knew was possible.

I've been using the tools of Access Consciousness® since 2012. I've used them to change the things I thought I could never change. I've gained a level of trust in myself and in my awareness that surpasses anything I could have imagined. These tools are pure magic and I can't wait to share them with you!

Cheers to going beyond our stories, into the creation of a new reality based on possibilities!

Patty Alfonso

Access Consciousness® Certified Facilitator
Creator Pole Dancing For Consciousness™
Creator The Essence of You™

PART I

LIFE BEFORE 30

HOW IT ALL BEGAN...

When I perceive the energy of the younger me, beyond the energy my family was choosing, I get the sense of total freedom, joy, exuberance and ease with my body and my being.

I remember dancing all of the time. Dancing all around the house, at restaurants and in school. I loved to dance. My body loved to move and I didn't care what anyone thought.

Does any child truly care what others are thinking? Do they just be and have fun? That was me!

I was 3 years old when my family decided that there was something wrong with me. They decided that I was a problem that needed to be fixed. I was one of those kids who couldn't sit still. I never did what I was told and I always said the things no one wanted me to say. In essence, everything I did was wrong.

Eventually, I started to believe that there *was* something wrong with me. I made myself small enough to fit into a tiny little box where I could hide from everyone around me. I even began hiding from myself. This way of being, of hiding, became what was normal to me.

I decided that if I could hide me and just be what everyone else wanted me to be, that everything would be ok. The problem was that no matter how much I hid, no matter how small I made myself, I was still the problem that needed to be fixed. The crazy one. The black sheep.

All I wanted, even at that age, was for everyone to be happy. To have fun. When people asked me what I wanted to be when I grew up, my answer was "Happy!"

Of course, that reply was not what anyone was looking for and most certainly nothing anyone could comprehend.

I was definitely the crazy, weird one in my family.

THIS IS WHAT I REMEMBER...

My father had a temper. My mother was controlling and thought the world was out to get her. My sister was given the job of making sure I didn't do anything wrong.

I remember being pushed away every time I tried to hug my Dad. I remember having the sense that he was uncomfortable around me.

I remember waking up in the middle of the night to my parents fighting. My dad was breaking things while my mom watched, stone faced, smoking a cigarette.

I remember that look my mother would give us if we were doing something that embarrassed her. The look that said: "You're gonna get it when we get home."

I remember being thrown down the stairs because I didn't feel like taking a bath that night.

I remember sharing a room with my sister, waking up in the middle of the night to our door opening and a figure coming into our room.

I remember visiting my aunt in Miami over the summer and going to the movies. Following her rules and being judged for just being a messy kid.

I remember our annual trip to the Tamiami Park Fair eating cotton candy and avoiding roller coasters at all cost. I didn't ride my first roller coaster until I was 21!

I remember trips on our boat to the Virgin Islands with friends.

I remember being told I was 'boy crazy' and that I'd be beautiful when I grew up.

I remember kindergarten, some of the 3rd and 4th grade, a few moments during my 5th and 6th grade, a trip to Europe during the summer between 8th and 9th grade and getting caught losing my virginity when I was 16.

I remember being the loud mouth in the family. Being aware of the energy below the surface of what was being said or done.

I remember everyone thought I was a handful and how wrong I felt for just being me.

WALKING-IN...

My childhood is a bit of a blur. I have some clear memories and some things my body remembers. None of my memories are complete, they're just snippets that come and go.

I used to think this was a problem. In this reality, some would say I have a dissociative disorder caused by traumatic experiences.

Thanks to the tools of Access Consciousness® I know that I'm a walk-in and I used to have multiple occupants.

A walk-in occurs when the Being occupying the body is done living here and chooses to leave - one Being walks out and the other walks-in.

The original Being can either leave or stay with the body. When the original Being stays then the body becomes a multiple occupant...one body, many beings.

The first time I remember walking in, I was in junior high. I remember suddenly appearing at a meeting. It was like I had just woken up and I was just there.

I looked around and couldn't recognize anyone or anything. I had no clue what I was doing there. Suddenly, the teacher called on me. I was frozen like a deer caught in the headlights.

As she spoke, I realized that not only had I been there before, but apparently I was the Secretary of this club. I don't even remember what kind of club it was!

Jump cut to me sitting on a bench in school wondering how the heck I had gotten there. I was so confused at the time.

And that's it. Memory ends. This is how I recall most of my childhood. In and out. In and out.

Makes it very interesting when my family asks me if I remember something we shared at some point. I just smile and nod and say yes and let them tell me the story.

Walk-ins are actually quite normal. It's just not something that we're taught in this reality.

NUMBING OUT...

I started drinking, smoking weed and having sex when I was 16. The memories I have become a bit more clear for me around this time in my life.

I remember deciding that 16 was a perfectly reasonable age to start having sex and doing drugs.

I got caught having sex with my boyfriend and my mother threatened to send me off to Japan. Given her reaction you would think I had committed bloody murder. Of course I thought these were completely normal teenage choices. I do remember being so mortified I wanted to die.

My mother and I had a difference of opinion about everything and I spent most of my high school years grounded for one indiscretion or another.

I had a sense of what worked for me about what I was choosing. Then there was my family's reality – their judgments and points of views about my choices. Somewhere along the way, I started buying into their reality. I started buying into the question that was impelled at me at most of the time:

"What is wrong with you?"

I could not get anything right. My grades weren't good

enough, my choices in men weren't good enough and my friends weren't good enough.

I was the family's go-to pain in the ass.

Things were a little easier for me when my sister went off to college. I had a wee bit more freedom since I didn't have a constant guardian on my back all the time.

THE COLLEGE YEARS...

Juilliard is a very prestigious dramatic arts school in New York and it was my dream to attend. My parents had the point of view that they did not want to send me off to a big college in a big city. So, my first choice was out of the question and I complied with their wishes.

My options for which college I could attend were limited to small colleges in the southern region of the US. My parents had the opinion that people are nicer in the south and therefore I would be safer.

I had gone to visit my sister at her college. It was a junior college 30 minutes west of Atlanta, GA. We spent the weekend partying and I figured this would be a fun place to go.

Not my smartest choice. The policing began again as my sister was given the job of making sure I didn't fuck up. I get this must have been hard on her. I was not easy to control.

The town the College was in was so small it wasn't even on the map. There was nothing to do over the weekends and we all spent most of our time high and drunk.

It was during my last year at this school, on my birthday, that I got drunk and decided to go see the boy I liked. We talked for a bit and I passed out on his bed. I woke up when he was on top of me, inside of me. I pushed him off and rolled over to go back to sleep.

When I woke up, I quietly crept out of the room. I knew something was not right as I left. I had the vague memory of what had happened. I also knew that I had chosen to show up drunk in the middle of the night.

He tried to speak to me about it at the next party, but I preferred to pretend nothing had happened. I never spoke to him again after that. It was years before I would admit to myself that I had never actually said yes to sex that night.

I remember crying when I was told I'd be graduating with my class. I was one of two from my group of friends that actually graduated on schedule.

I received my Associates Degree and went on to get my Bachelors Degree in Sociology.

During college, per the insistence of my family, I traded my dreams for a degree. There was no acting and the only dancing I did was on top of bars at clubs.

THE GIFTS OF BEING A NANNY...

During my junior year of college I became a nanny. I stayed with this family for 9 years. Being with this family saved my life. Literally.

I went from a family that did not trust me, thought I was crazy, wanted to disown me and cut me off to a family that trusted me with their children and their home. They took me on family vacations, invited me to live with them and cared for me in a way I had never been cared for.

The Rabinowitz's taught me about true caring, gratitude, trust, honor and allowance. I was allowed to be me. No matter what it looked like. And it was ok.

This was probably the first time in my life where everything I did was right! The way I was with the kids, the way I helped out around the house, even my cooking skills were appreciated!

When I first started working there, we went to Synagogue for dinner. At the time, I knew nothing about what being an Orthodox Jew was all about. I had a nose ring and a pink streak in my hair. I showed up for work in cut-off jeans and a tank top. And yet, without apologies or embarrassment, we went to dinner at the Synagogue. Being around Mrs.

Rabinowitz always made me feel comfortable. She didn't shame me or ask me to change.

She truly accepted me as I was and never asked for anything different.

Mr. Rabinowitz was the loving father I never had. He was kind to his children, loved his family and loved coming home. I was always impressed to see him helping out around the house. I don't think I ever saw him get angry.

I remember the first time he gave me a hug. As an Orthodox Jewish married man, you are not allowed to touch other women besides your wife. And when he hugged me, I felt cared for and loved. It was the first time a father figure had ever truly held me.

It was with this family that I began to see myself differently. I became aware of the ways in which I could perceive energy and choose based on that.

Once I was helping Mrs. Rabinowitz get ready for Shabbos Dinner and one of her guests had arrived early. We were all in the kitchen and Mrs. Arnovitz acknowledged the ease with which I moved around Mrs. Rabinowitz and seemed to know what was required before she asked me for it. She wished she could find someone like me to help her around the house.

Another time, I took the boys to visit Mrs. Rabinowitz at the hospital. She was recovering from a pretty major surgery and she looked quite frail. I looked over at her oldest son. Instinctively I went over to let him know she was ok and he didn't have to worry. I had perceived what was happening in his universe and said what was required to soothe him.

They brought out in me the caring, loving, fun, kind kid that had always been there. Being with them healed something in me that I barely have words for. At the time, I knew I was re-living my childhood with this family and re-wiring my neurological pathways.

My time working with them allowed me to step out of the little box I had been living in. It was a small step and a beginning.

But it didn't last long.

BEYOND FAMILY...

Once I completed College and got my degree, I declared that I had done what my parents wanted me to do and now it was time to do what I wanted to do.

I promptly began taking acting classes, going on auditions, working and looking at what I really wanted out of life. I even took ballet lessons! Creativity wasn't valued in my family, so I began exploring what was creative for me and made me happy.

Besides telling people I wanted to be happy when I grew up, I would also tell them that I wanted to be a cross between Marilyn Monroe and Mother Theresa.

Of course people thought I was cute when I said it...but I meant it!

I had no clue what that would look, like but I began working on the Marilyn Monroe phase of my life. I figured, if I could get famous, people would listen to me and I would be able to change the world. This was one of the things I knew I wanted out of life. I wanted to help people. I wanted people to be happy and have joy.

I spent 10 years in Atlanta, GA. I built up my acting resume and my acting reel with the target of someday moving to Los Angeles.

I met a boy. I fell in love and moved across the country to live with him in San Francisco.

At the time, it seemed a great first step to getting to Los Angeles. I didn't know anyone in LA and due to my very controlled, sheltered upbringing, moving to a huge city where I knew no one was a scary thought.

We had agreed that we would spend some time in the Bay Area and then we would move to LA together. I would continue to build my acting skills, get an agent and then move to LA with more ease.

Well, the boy was not my best choice. He turned out to be as abusive as my father, as controlling as my mother and an even greater police officer than my sister!

We ended things and went our separate ways. Of course, my original plan had worked, in a way. I did build up my resume and get an agent who referred me to one of the best agencies in Los Angeles.

I arrived in Los Angeles single, ahead of the game and quite pleased with myself!

SHUTTING DOWN, LOCKING UP AND WAKING UP...

For the first 27 years of my life I became really comfortable hiding in order to please those who felt uncomfortable around me. I hid behind drugs, alcohol, parties and abusive relationships.

As I look back now, I am aware that the more I chose for my family, the more I hid in order to please everyone else. The more I pleased others, the more I shut myself down.

For years, I shut off my desires, my awarenesses, my body and my being. I gave myself up completely in order to please everyone else around me. This would become a pattern I had to learn to break in order to be free and happy.

Eventually, shutting down began to be reflected through my body. Before I got to energy healing, I was in total lock down.

My body did not move with ease in the world and there was an overall sadness that permeated everything. I was stiff, numb and miserable.

I cut myself off from life and the expression of it through my body. Relationships, work, sex, play – everything was dull. I shut out the awarenesses that my body was capable of giving me in order to not be present with other people's judgments of me.

Even then, in the stupor created by drugs and alcohol, I knew I was slowly dying.

I had a little voice in my head that kept telling me I would die if I kept choosing this life. I would not create what I came here to create.

About a year after I began hearing this voice, I made the demand to awaken my senses again, no matter what it took, no matter what I lost and no matter what I had to change.

I knew I had something special to gift to this world and I would not leave without expressing that gift.

My time in Los Angeles, CA was a huge part in my journey towards finding me and going beyond my family.

THE END OF THE BEGINNING...

I spent 14 years in Los Angeles.

These years were a long journey of self-discovery, self-mastery and healing. I worked at various small businesses over the years always making time for auditions and acting work.

I created an amazing group of friends in the industry.

I was in a soap opera, acted in commercials, independent films, did some extra work and collaborated on lots of small projects. As time went by, acting no longer spoke to me.

My Marilyn Monroe plan was not panning out the way I had imagined. I was in an industry that judged everything about me. I was too pretty, too short, not Latin enough, not white enough, not tall enough, not slutty enough....not the best environment for someone recovering from the wrongness of being!

I drank more. I did more drugs. I created more abusive relationships. All of which led me to seek the healing arts.

I began working with a healer on a weekly basis and became aware that it was time to work on the Mother Theresa part of my master plan to change the world! Cute. I'm very cute!

I spent 4 years at the Lionheart Institute for Transpersonal Energy Healing. I became certified as a Body/Mind Counselor and an Energy Healing Therapist. I let go of acting, got sober and began my own business as a healer and a life coach.

It was during my time there that I recall having another walk-in experience.

We were learning a new healing technique that was designed to encourage us to establish our boundaries with the therapist.

We were to clearly and loudly claim our "No!" several times. Very quickly the room became a shouting match of men and women claiming their "No!" to their healers.

Some turned into "Don't touch me!". Others turned into "Get away from me!". I was triggered immediately. There was a lot of energetic releasing of crossed boundaries throughout many lifetimes for everyone.

While I was on the healing table, I went into tetany. Tetany is the involuntary contraction of muscles. I lost complete control of my body. My stomach was undulating while my hands and face were frozen. I was awake and aware and scared.

My healers stood with me, comforted me and encouraged me to stay present. As I slowly let go of total control, my body softened and I was able to experience the muscle contractions with more ease.

After the healing was complete, I got up and went outside

for some fresh air. Everything was different. There was a clarity in my universe I had never had before. I could perceive energy on a whole new level. I could actually see the molecules in the sky vibrating with energy and forming the Flower of Life pattern. It was amazing.

I went home and fell asleep. The next day, I awoke and everything was different again. Everything was slower. I felt as if I was learning to use my body again. I could hear every sound so clearly. I could really feel my body and I could feel my being in my body.

Shortly after that, I began working with the school. I had gotten so much out of the tools they taught that I knew I wanted to be a part of bringing those tools into the world.

I used all the skills I had learned from working in small business and combined them with my new skills as a healer to expand the school.

There was so much I wanted to contribute to the school. I also wanted to teach and create workshops. Finally, the Mother Theresa part of my plan was kicking in!

During my time there I met an amazing business coach, Carolyn McCormick, who introduced me to the tools that changed my life forever – the tools of Access Consciousness®.

She had previously worked with Anthony Robbins and used her expertise to help me expand my private practice. I had my own office and private coaching clients. I began creating and facilitating my own workshops and having the dream life I had always known was possible.

And then, as things usually do, something changed. I was bored. Nothing was going as fast as I knew I could be going.

I was not creating as much as I knew I could create.

And I knew it was time to move on...to a new beginning.

ACKNOWLEDGING WHAT I CREATED...

Dr. Dain Heer, one of the Co-Creators of Access Consciousness®, came up with a lovely little acronym for Family.

I was shocked when I first heard this and, with time, it has actually saved me from buying into the lies of who my family thinks I am. This little acronym created so much space for me around family and the choices we were all making.

> **F**ucked-up
> **A**nd
> **M**ainly
> **I**nterested in
> **L**imiting
> **Y**ou

Gary Douglas, the Co-Creator of Access Consciousness® says that we choose our families because we know they can never stop us.

These two things are both true for me. I am incredibly grateful for everything I created with my family. Every choice has led me to right now and right now is pretty fuckin' awesome.

During a private session with a Facilitator, I was able to

see and acknowledge that I had created myself as the black sheep of the family. My choices had led to that creation.

The moment I let go of the story that being the black sheep was something that was imposed and perpetrated *on* me, I was able to change the way I view my history.

As I write this, I've become acutely aware that the more I chose for my family, the more I withdrew from myself and what I desired to create in my life. Those were my choices.

When I was really young, I didn't care what they thought. I chose for myself and, even though I was grounded for most of my teenage years, I was happy. I didn't get their ways and I didn't really care.

Then, I started caring about what they thought about me and what they wanted from me. This choice led me to give up on being ME. I chose that! They didn't make me give up. I chose it.

And, on that same note, everything I have chosen has gotten me to right now. As I said before, right now is pretty awesome. Had I not experienced what I created, most of my life would not exist!

Allowing other people's points of views to influence my choices is a pattern I'm still working on letting go of. I get stuck in trying to be perfect, being liked and pleasing other people.

Some would say those are my life lessons...I say I'm changing that now.

PART II

A New Beginning

The Magic of Pole Dancing

Have you ever walked in the rain and allowed it to caress every inch of your skin?

Have you ever eaten anything that exploded in your mouth and expanded every cell in your body?

Have you ever gotten dressed and felt so good that everyone you talked to that day complemented you?

What about dancing? Have you ever just allowed your body to move the way it wants to move? Not trying to do anything, just being the dance?

It took me over half of my life to be able to say yes to these questions. As a matter of fact, if you had asked me these questions years ago I would not have known what you meant at all!

One of the requirements at my energy healing school was to find a form of movement or exercise that we could add to our daily self-care routine.

I was already doing yoga, kickboxing and Pilates. I did the occasional walk and run as well. None of these made my body very happy.

I began asking questions because I knew there was

something else possible. I made the demand to awaken my senses again, no matter what it took.

One of the first things to show up in my life was pole dancing. For the first time my body was happy again.

I began my journey with pole dancing in 2011.

I could tell you that when I first heard about pole dancing, I was shocked at the idea of stripping as a way of working out.

That would be a total lie though.

My body practically leapt at the chance to pole dance. So much so that when I was looking for belly dancing classes, she actually led me to a pole dancing studio instead. Smart body...

I remember going to a strip club in college. I was in awe of the women who were working there. The way they sashayed their bodies across the stage, the way men lusted after them, the beauty in their curves and the softness of their skin glistening in the lights.

They seemed to be so free with their bodies. I wanted that. Of course, I couldn't have that. What would everyone think?

Fifteen years later I found myself in a candlelit dance studio with a group of women.

Sitting around a pole, music playing softly in the background, I claimed my desire to re-connect to my feminine essence.

I explained that somewhere along my journey I have shut down my body and it was destroying my life.

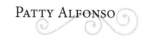

That night changed my life forever.

What I have gained since has been beyond anything I could have imagined. Over the years, I have learned to listen to my body and be present with her in a whole new way.

Pole dancing gifted me with the chance to let go of my mind and surrender to her.

Surrendering to the way she wants to move, the music she wants to dance to, the moves she wants to make. No matter what they look like!

This didn't happen overnight though. There were many times when I noticed my mind did not want to trust or honor the intelligence of my body.

My mind would say:

> "You want me to do what with just one hand?"
> "I'm not strong enough to hold myself upside down!"
> "Ok, that is crazy, I can't do that!"
> "You should not be touching yourself like that"

Musings and lies created by the mind...

There were certain tricks that absolutely required knowing my body would support me and take care of me.

There were so many times when I let go and she surprised me with total delight.

There were other times when I listened to her and chose to do the trick some other time.

Pole dancing was about tuning in to my body and allowing

her to choose what she required in that moment. It was about honoring where she was that day and choosing for her, not against her.

And then, there were the women in my class...the beautiful, courageous women who were on this journey with me. We clapped, cheered and supported each other. We celebrated everything. Nothing was a failure.

How can anything be a failure when you're honoring you?

Pole dancing wasn't the only thing that contributed to my transformation.

In 2012, I began adding the tools I was learning in Access Consciousness® to my dances.

I was aware that there were things locked into my body that were being released through my dancing.

As you've read, over the years my body had picked up judgments, projections and expectations and shut herself down from the cruelties of this reality.

All of that was unwinding and I was finally alive. In this body. In this life. Creating and generating beyond anything I could have imagined.

None of this would have been possible if I hadn't included my body on this journey towards consciousness.

In my universe, pole dancing is an invitation to more consciousness with your body *and* your being.

In my universe, pole dancing and Access Consciousness®

have merged into a delicious adventure where I get to explore more of the Being I truly be...beyond the judgments and projections.

THE TOOLS THAT CHANGED MY LIFE

I knew there was more to be opened within me. In this wonderful reality there is always more to be explored. When you have the courage to do so.

Using the tools of Access Consciousness®, I became aware of the barriers I was using to block everyone out.

I became aware that the only place I was allowing myself to express my sexualness was in my pole dancing class.

What would it take to be this space all of the time? The space of being present with my body. The space of having pleasure and joy with my body beyond the candlelit classroom.

Ask and you shall receive...Tantra came into my life. Charu, my tantra teacher, held a beautiful space for me to begin exploring what was pleasurable to me.

Turned out, after all this time, I had no idea what pleasure was or how to have it!

The tantric exercises facilitated a deeper opening of my body and the release of all the energy I was locking into my body.

It also created more awareness of who I was being in my relationship and the things that I needed to change in order for me to be happy.

I became aware that if I didn't know what was pleasurable to me I couldn't expect my partner to know either.

Out in the world I was stuck. The energy I was projecting stated "If you come near me I will kill you". At one point in my life this was necessary. It was what I had created in order to feel safe in the world.

My life experiences included all forms of abuse – verbal, sexual, financial and spiritual. And then there was the abuse I was trying to heal in the women in my family. And the lifetimes of abuse we have all been through.

I was aware of all of it and my body was protecting against it. The thing is, when you resist something it actually persists in your life. All I was really doing was creating more abuse. More separation. More judgment.

The more I chose to hide from abuse, the more I created it. I didn't want to be aware of all the abuse in the world so I kept myself shut down.

Imagine what it would be like to have so much awareness that you can perceive the energy of a situation and instinctively know if you need to remove yourself from that situation.

There have been times when I can perceive someone has the intention of hurting me in some way. The level of awareness I am willing to have now takes care of me. I trust myself.

It wasn't always like that; there were many times in my life when I didn't trust myself. A time when everyone around me accused me of being selfish and crazy and I allowed those accusations to define me.

Being in Access Consciousness® gave me more of me – because I chose it. I chose to have more of me *for* me. That sense that I was a gift to this world and there was something special I had come here to do kept pushing me to choose more.

What good was I doing by hiding? What would I facilitate in the world if I didn't step out into it?

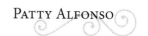

THE QUESTION THAT CHANGED EVERYTHING ...AGAIN

Do you have anyone in your life that is in total allowance of you?

Anyone who adores you and cares for you without judgment? No matter what you choose?

For me, those people are Gary Douglas and Dain Heer, the co-founders of Access Consciousness®.

I began showing up to all the classes I could take. Their complete allowance for me to show up was remarkable. The caring, generosity, vulnerability, honoring, creativity and healing they chose inspired me to truly embody all of me. No matter what it looked like.

During a private session with Dain, he asked me a question that would change my life forever:

What if there is nothing wrong with you?

WHAT? It tweaked my Universe, as I had been believing my entire life that there was something wrong with me! Even after all the healing I had done, there was still an underlying current within me that kept me looping back to me being wrong.

As I continued to ask myself this question, I became aware that what I believed was my greatest wrongness - the ability to see and say what no one else could see and say - was actually my greatest strongness.

And so I began asking myself:

If there is nothing wrong with me, what would I like to create?

No one had ever asked me what I desired to create. As much as I had stepped out of my tiny little box, there was still a big part of me in there.

I may have had better role models, but I was still basing a lot of my choices on what other people wanted me to be and do.

I was still giving up myself to please everyone around me. Giving up myself in order to fit in. Giving up myself so that everyone around me would be happy.

This question opened up a new world of possibilities for me and I began creating my life the way I had always known was possible.

And then, in 2012 I created the business that had been hiding deep within me for lifetimes.

I took the things that brought me and my body the most joy and I put them together to create something that didn't exist in this reality.

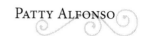

Pole Dancing For Consciousness™ became an invitation to a new way of being with the world for everyone who chose it...including myself.

This creation was a huge step out of my tiny little box to a global business with clients from all over the world.

THE BASICS IN ACCESS CONSCIOUSNESS®

There are so many Access Consciousness® tools I could tell you about!

This body of work is one of the most inclusive and expansive bodies of work I've ever played with in my career.

You can apply these tools to change anything and they are designed to "Empower you to know that you know®".

I'd like to give you some of the basics so you can get started right away.

And, the rest of the sections will make more sense if you have these first!

ASKING QUESTIONS AND MAKING DIFFERENT CHOICES

Gary and Dain talk about always being in the question.

The mind can only create based on what it already knows. When we function from our minds, we can only create based on our past experiences.

If those past experiences had created what you desired... would you be here right now? I know I would still be hiding in my little tiny box!

"No problem can be solved from the same level of consciousness that created it."
~Albert Einstein

Questions open the door to new possibilities. They open the door to new choices that weren't available in your limited mind.

When you ask a question without seeking "the right answer," you allow the Universe to show you the unimaginable that goes beyond the mind.

Here are my two favorite questions to ask:

What else is possible?®

How does it get any better than this? ™

The key here is to open the door to *new* possibilities and to expand the energy beyond the mind and into the gifts the Universe is just waiting to give you.

As you begin to ask questions, you'll notice the universe will begin providing new possibilities. Then, it is time to make different choices.

Every time you make a different choice, new possibilities will get created. Then you ask more questions, and make new choices!

"Every time you choose something, you get closer to the reality you desire to create." ~Gary Douglas

If you are in the adventure of creating something new in your life, it can actually be quite fun!

Throughout the rest of the book and in the Practical Tools for Pragmatic Change section, I will be giving you lots of questions you can play with right away.

FOLLOWING THE ENERGY

When you begin to ask questions, you have to follow the energy of what is light and expansive for **you**.

When you choose based on the energy of something, rather than your cognitive conclusions, you begin to invite the magic that is available in the universe to create *with* you.

What is light and expansive is <u>true</u> for you.

What is heavy and a contraction is <u>not true</u> for you.

Choosing what is light and expansive will always create more for you than choosing based on your mind.

Before using these tools, I would choose things that would make others happy. I would choose things because other people wanted me to choose them. I had created a life that everyone else approved of but I was miserable!

When I began following the energy, I learned that the Universe always has my back. I learned to trust myself and my awareness. I learned that I am so different from everyone around me.

I was able to see me and my capacities and honor what worked for me, beyond what other people wanted for me. I truly began to live *my* life.

Are you willing to perceive the energy of what will create more for you? Are you willing to make that demand for you?

"If you want to find the secrets of the Universe, think in terms of energy, frequency and vibration."

~ Nikola Tesla

KNOWING WHO YOU TRULY BE

In my journey towards rediscovering the essence of me, I had to look at every single point of view, judgment, conclusion and decision I had ever made about myself and everyone around me.

Every time I had a thought, feeling or emotion I would ask these questions:

Who does this belong to?®
Who am I being?

I obsessively looked at everything that went through my awareness and slowly peeled off the layers of projections and expectations I had been living from to find what was truly me.

I had bought my family's points of view as if they were mine. I would behave the way my mother, father or sister would behave in situations.

I had no sense of what was true for me until I began using these questions to clear the energy and open up to the true essence of me.

Today, I continue to ask these questions and create myself anew every day. Everyday is a new adventure in finding out who I desire to be and opening up to the glorious adventures of life and living.

When you are truly being you, when you trust you and you know you have your own back, the Universe can support you in creating anything you desire.

People can show up in your life that actually desire to contribute to you. Everything in your life can change for the better....it always does. You have to choose *you* first though!

This conversation is partly about you being you. It's also about creating you every day - beyond the decisions, judgments, conclusions and computations that you have made about who you are and who you're supposed to be.

Allowing yourself to change at a moment's notice and choose something different creates a world of freedom for you and everyone around you.

*Who do you want to
choose to be today?*

*What would you like
to create today?*

JUDGMENT KILLS POSSIBILITIES

Judgment is the greatest killer of possibilities here in this reality. The moment you judge something as good or bad, you're cutting off the gifts you could receive.

We are taught to judge from a very young age. This is right. That is wrong. This is good. That is bad. You're supposed to live your life according to these judgments.

My family judged as a form of love. Only when I did what they thought was right and correct did they love and approve of me.

When I was doing something they judged as wrong and incorrect, then I was the problem that needed to be fixed.

A judgment is someone's point of view based on their past experiences, projections andexpectations.

What if everything was just an *interesting* point of view?

What if everything was just a choice? And those choices created different outcomes? And every outcome was a possibility rather than a wrongness or a consequence?

When I was young, I never really got why I couldn't just

do whatever worked for me. In my world, as long as I was choosing what worked for me it would create more for everyone else around me. As they say, if you're happy everyone is happy!

To me, there was no right or wrong. Just choices. Choices that created different paths to be traveled.

Of course, in my family all of my choices had "consequences that I had to face." Is that light and expansive? Or heavy and a contraction?

Your point of view creates your reality. If you are always judging yourself, your body or your choices, what do you perceive you are creating with all of that judgment?

If you had no judgment about what this journey is supposed to look like and there was no right or wrong, what other possibilities would be available?

We make all of these decisions and conclusions based on our judgment about what things are supposed to be like. We end up blocking all of the other possibilities that are available because of those decisions.

Would you be willing to destroy all of the decisions, judgments and conclusions you've created in order for new possibilities to show up?

APPLYING THE TOOLS TO YOUR BODY

You can apply all of these tools to create more communion with your body as well.

You can start by asking your body questions in regards to what your body desires.

You can follow the energy of what is light and true for you and your body. Every body is different. What is yummy for you may not be yummy for others!

We sometimes override what our bodies desire in favor of what we desire. And, at other times, what is light for our bodies does not make any sense to our logical mind.

You actually create your body based on your judgments of your body.

I met a woman once who was in her early 40's. She had 9 children and had been pregnant for most of her marriage. She also had the cutest, sweet little body and a great figure.

Later I learned that she loved being pregnant. It gave her and her body joy. So, did she create her body based on that joy? I would say so!

What else is possible with your body you haven't imagined yet?

*If you had no judgments about your body,
would that create more ease in your life?*

If you allowed your body to show you what it desires, what would that create?

In the next section we'll be diving deep into this topic.

For now, let's explore awakening, embodying and unleashing the magnificence of having a body!

WHAT IS IT TO EMBODY ANYWAY?

I had to ask this question a lot when I first came to Access, as I really had no clue what this meant.

Let's explore this a little further, shall we?

What would it take to enjoy your body?

What if you allowed your body to contribute to you?

What if every molecule in your body could vibrate with orgasmic energy?

Sounds kinda fun this whole embodiment thing doesn't it?

To me, embodiment is being in communion with my body. Embodiment is the willingness to hear what my body is saying and surrender to it. Joyful embodiment is allowing your body to contribute orgasmically to your life.

There are so many fun things we can only do in this reality with a body! Could you get a massage if you didn't have a body? Would you be able to dance? Have sex? Eat? Caress a lover?

In the following sections, we'll dive deep into embodiment. We'll explore the ways we can surrender to the consciousness of our bodies.

We'll play with the different possibilities available with our bodies and ask lots of questions!

During my first Energetic Synthesis of Being class with Dr. Dain Heer in Venice, Italy, I had a taste of joyful embodiment and it changed my life.

Here's a sweet little story for you that I like to call:

Here Comes the Rain Again...

An Orgasmic Walk through Venice

It was about 4am when I woke up and heard the rain falling outside my window. I thought to myself: "Dammit...I was going to straighten my hair today." I slipped back into a cozy slumber as I heard the raindrops gently kissing the earth.

I rose at 7:30am...Still raining...sigh...

Ok, well...How does it get better than this?™

First day of Access Consciousness'® Energetic Synthesis of Being with Dr. Dain Heer. Yay! How does it get any better than this?™

I was in Italy after all.

I started getting ready and my mind began to wander... "I have a long walk to the venue and no umbrella"...

I began asking questions...

"What else is possible?®

My body chose what it desired to wear ... "I could take a

water bus...hmmm...that feels heavy...what grand and glorious adventure can me and my body have today?"

I proceeded to put on my make-up... "I could buy an umbrella on the way...what can I receive from the rain today?"

I did my hair..."What would it take for nature to do my hair today?"

As I walked down the stairs from my apartment to the cobblestone alley, my body began to buzz with excitement.

I stepped outside and felt the cold drops of rain on my head. A tingle went down my spine all the way through my legs and back into the Earth.

Wow...In that moment I chose to let Nature have her way with me. No need for waterbuses or umbrellas. I was open to receiving what she had to offer.

More drops fell on my head, each one cold and refreshing, dripping down my scalp, through my hair. It felt delicious.

My body was so happy! My legs quivered as the rain caressed my body and I allowed her to gift to me. She was beautiful and kind and so generous.

I ran my fingers through my hair. My touch was filled with caring and gratitude. The sensation of my wet and dry hair between my fingers sent another rush of energy through my body. Oh my...

I expanded my energy out into the streets of Venice and then farther out into the Universe.

I became aware of other people's realities. Humans frustrated with the rain, cursing her for getting them wet.

"Hmmm...That's an interesting point of view." If only they could step into my reality and just allow her to kiss them.

One can only invite people to choose something different. I chose again to be with the rain.

"Wow...How does it get any better than this?^{TM}"

My body let me know she wanted some rain on her neck. I dropped my head, moved my hair and walked under an awning that was dripping with rain.

I allowed the raindrops to fall on my neck. Oh my...shivers went down my spine and through my legs back into Earth again. I had created my own reality with the rain. She was talking to me, touching me the way a lover would and I was quivering with joy and delight.

I tossed my hair back and the sweet, cold air gently made love to my face. For a moment my mind interrupted me and I worried about my make up. That lasted about 10 seconds and I chose again to be with the rain.

My entire body buzzed with the orgasmic energy I had been asking for since I went to the 7 Day event in Costa Rica. I could sense my heart beating, the blood running through my veins in a way I had never felt before and it was glorious!

As I approached the San Marco Square I noticed everyone avoiding the rain. My body wanted to strut across the

Square and continue this marvelous experience so I went for it.

"Wow...how does it get any better than this?!"

I arrived at class and the greeter acknowledged that I was the happiest person to walk through the door.

I was buzzing, shaking, happy, joyful, excited, turned on and oh, so grateful for my orgasmic walk through Venice with the rain.

What would it take for you to allow the rain to make love to you?

I think the room was a little crooked when I walked in...and by the way, my hair looked amazing for the rest of the day.

This is what it *can* look like to use the tools with your body and enjoy your body.

Let's play with some of the tools that I've used with myself and my clients to have more joy!

PART III

YOUR BODY & THE ELEMENTS OF INTIMACY

YOUR BODY & THE ELEMENTS OF INTIMACY

Being disconnected from my body for most of my life was fertile ground for the growth and expansion that choosing more communion would create.

Before I began my work with Pole Dancing For Consciousness™ and Access Consciousness®, I did not communicate with my body at all. I did not experience any kind of sensations with my body.

The taste of food was dull, my body was numb and I didn't enjoy being touched or hugged. I would push my body to do things that she did not enjoy because I thought it was the right thing to do. There was rigidity in my body that created a stiffness in the way I walked. It was not fun for me to have a body at all!

I was functioning from the head up. Aimlessly wandering around thinking...and thinking....and thinking....and mostly, confusing myself. Functioning from the various insane thoughts my mind generated based on my life experiences.

I was hiding behind the barriers I had created in order to keep myself "safe" from the perceived harshness of the world.

What if your body can contribute to you in more ways that you could have ever imagined?

When I first learned about the Elements of Intimacy, I started applying them to my relationships. I quickly realized that I didn't know what is was to have intimacy with myself or with my body. And, if I did not know what this was for me, how could I have it with someone else?

I started playing with these elements and discovered what it would be like to have them with myself and with my body, and then it became a lot easier to have them with other people.

The Access Consciousness® Elements of Intimacy are:

1. Gratitude

2. Allowance

3. Trust

4. Honor

5. Vulnerability

HAVING AND BEING GRATITUDE

When I first started looking at this and looking at the wisdom that my body has, I couldn't help but step into the space of gratitude.

What does being grateful for your body look like for you?

The body has its own innate brilliance. For example, did you know that every cell in your body knows exactly what its "job" is from the moment it's conceived?

Be with that for a moment...every cell knows what it's going to be and do in your body from the moment it is conceived in the womb.

Have you ever noticed that your body breathes on it's own? Your heart beats? Your blood flows? Your body knows when it has to go to the bathroom or when it requires food. Your body functions without YOU having to DO anything.

Your body *knows*.

Throughout the body's lifetime, all the cells, organs, systems that keep your body alive know what to do. You, the being, are the energy that keeps it all together. You are the space between the molecules that has created this magnificent body.

Isn't that amazing?

When I perceive the energy of my body and all it does for itself and for me, I can't help but be grateful for her.

Your heart *knows* that it's going to pump and it's going to circulate blood through your entire body. Your white blood cells *know* that they are there to fend off sickness.

When I truly received this knowing about my body, I became so much more aware of the magic that my body is, her capacities and the wisdom that she knows.

This allowed me to step into this space of "Oh my gosh thank you, thank you for breathing, thank you for us waking up this morning and being able to enjoy this beautiful day!"

Remember the family I worked for during my college years? While I was with them I learned a lot about being an Orthodox Jew.

Besides being completely fascinated by their commitment to their life, I was also totally curious about everything they did on a daily basis. Good thing they were always open to answering all of my questions!

One day I was at their house and I bumped into one of the girls coming out of the bathroom. I noticed she was murmuring something to herself. I asked her what she was doing, she said she was praying. This is how that conversation went:

"Huh? Praying? How come?"

"Yeah" she said, "you pray and you give thanks that everything worked while you were in the bathroom."

That moment changed something in me about my body and the miracles that are being created every time I take a breath.

Do you take your body for granted?

Have you ever stubbed your toe or your thumb and all of a sudden you can't use it for a few days? Then you become aware of how much you do use it?

Do you judge your body?

In an Access Consciousness® Body Class I learned that cellulite shows up when we are judging something about our bodies. When I find cellulite on my body, I ask: "What am I judging about myself? What am I judging about my body?

Then I do my best to step into a little bit more gratitude for my body and the cellulite actually disappears, which I think is quite phenomenal.

Thank you body for that capacity.

BEING IN ALLOWANCE OF YOUR BODY

To have allowance with your body is to look at what she/he desires and have it all be an interesting point of view. Allowance is about not judging what your body prefers.

What if today, your body wanted to stay in bed and watch movies?

What if today, your body wanted to go outside and sit in the sun?

What if today, your body wanted to have a hamburger and French fries?

What if today, your body wanted to sit at your computer and work all day – without taking a break?

When you judge something as right or wrong, you are actually cutting off the energy of possibility from your life. Judgment is one of the biggest ways in which we choose to lock up our body's wisdom.

If nothing was the right thing to do and nothing was the wrong thing to do, everything would just be a choice that creates a new possibility. And this applies to your body as well!

Our bodies function from consciousness.

They don't have a point of view about what they look like, how big they are, how small they are or what they eat. Our bodies don't judge themselves! We judge them.

Once you start communicating with your body, you can start asking your body questions about what it desires.

The fun begins once your body actually starts giving you the energy of what it would likc!

And even more fun is being aware of the difference between what you like and what your body likes!

This brings us to the next element...

TRUSTING YOUR BODY

If you choose to have fun while exploring what your body prefers, you can begin to build trust between you and your body.

When you begin to ask your body questions *and* you begin to listen to what your body desires *and* choose for and with your body, you'll start to see that you can trust the consciousness of your body.

Your body functions *from* consciousness. It does not have all of the points of view and judgments that you The Being are holding onto.

When you let go of your points of view and allow your body to choose, greater possibilities can show up!

Trust is not blind faith. Trust is knowing what you need to do to care for you.

Does your body know what it needs to do to care for itself?

Do you allow your body to know? Or do you override your body with your judgments and points of view?

Would you be willing to trust the innate knowing of your body?

When I started taking pole dancing classes this element of trust was something that really came up for me. The teacher was showing us a particular trick and I had this awareness that I was really going to have to trust my body to do this trick. I had to really trust that my body knew in order to fully let go.

This trick was a spinning trick and we had to spin backwards and your leg would automatically hook onto the pole.

I was able to let go...and I flew with such delight! To this day, it's one of my favorite tricks to do on the pole!

I was recently working with a client and we were looking at the energy that came up for her around being in allowance of her body and trusting her body. The underlying energy was that she simply did not want to let go of control.

She was used to being in charge of everything in her life. She did not trust anyone to do anything for her and she always did everything for herself.

Trusting and being in allowance of her body brought up the energy of not trusting anyone else or herself. She wasn't willing to see that her body cared for her and that her body would have her back.

We took baby steps and started with acknowledging the times when she did allow her body to choose and whether it had created more or less for her in her life.

She talked about her body's capacity to choose the clothes it wanted to wear and how that always worked out well for her in the long run.

When she allowed her body to choose, and she trusted that awareness, it always worked out! There was more ease during her day. She didn't have to worry about what she was wearing or if it was going to get dirty or if she chose something that wasn't going to be appropriate. When she allowed her body to choose, it always fit, it worked with everything.

Would you be willing to be in allowance of your body?

To trust your body?

HONORING YOUR BODY

When you have allowance and trust, you can follow it with a bit of honor for your body.

When you honor your body, you treat her/him with regard and you recognize the miracle that it truly is. You see what is working for you and for your body and choose based on what your body would like no matter what anyone else's point of view is.

When you honor your body, you can recognize the miracle that it truly is. You can see what is working for you and for your body and choose based on that rather than based on what others think.

I have a few examples that may illustrate this with ease.

I used to smoke cigarettes when I was in college. I had quit smoking for quite a long time when I went to Venice, Italy.

I was going through a lot of changes and I started smoking again. At the time, it soothed my body and facilitated me through some of those changes. I asked my body and my body was ok with me smoking so I chose to give myself a year of smoking without judging myself for it.

After a year or so my body stopped enjoying it. I would feel tired, nauseous and sick after a cigarette and it was clear to me that my body was done. The thing was that I, the being, was still enjoying it! So I began to ask, "What else is possible?®" with smoking.

Shortly after I began to ask, I ended up getting introduced to vaping. When I first tried it, my body loved it and I was still able to have the sensation of smoking!

I honored my body. I honored what I desired and came up with something that worked for both of us.

When I chose pole dancing as my favorite way to move with my body, it brought up all kinds of judgments and projections from some of my family members. My sister even sent me some articles about how pole dancing leads to sex trafficking.

It didn't matter to me though. My body demanded it and I chose it. I followed the energy because I knew it would create something amazing for me and for my body.

It ended up creating a world-wide business for me and took me beyond anything I could have imagined!

When I go to the gym for Zumba or yoga, I'm that crazy girl in the front of the class doing whatever her body desires. If the Zumba routine is too fast and my body wants to move slower, I honor that. If the yoga pose is too hard on my body and she wants to adjust, I honor that.

What does honoring your body look like for you?

What choices can you make today that would honor your body right away?

What if you asked these questions every day, followed the energy and played with everything that shows up?

Remember, what is light is true for you. What is heavy is a lie.

How much fun can you have discovering the language of your body?

There's lot more questions to play with in the Practical Tools for Pragmatic Change section of this book!

BEING VULNERABLE WITH YOUR BODY

Being vulnerable with myself and with my body has been one of the greatest challenges and gifts I've encountered so far.

In my family, we were not allowed to be vulnerable. We always had to project that we were perfect when in actuality, below the surface of perfection; there was abuse, alcoholism, rage and fear. But we couldn't tell anyone that...

We never really had open conversations about anything. I attempted several times but, being the child that said what was not allowed, I was mostly in trouble for it.

Being vulnerable is never putting up barriers to anything.

Being vulnerable with your body is about being able to lower your barriers and perceive, know, be and receive anything that shows up. The good, the bad and the ugly...the magical, magnificent and annoying...All of it with no point of view, no judgment.

Being vulnerable with your body is about being willing to receive your body's requests, being able to perceive with your body and being totally present with your body no matter what is showing up.

"Hi cellulite, what's up? You're there, cool. I'm not going to put barriers up to you...what are you trying to tell me?"

That is vulnerability, just being with your body. Asking questions, staying present and receiving.

This reality projects that being vulnerable is being weak. This is not true. Being vulnerable takes a lot of courage. And when you are not putting up barriers to anything, you are able to be aware of everything.

Awareness is your greatest asset. With time and a great deal of practice, being vulnerable with my body allows me to include my body in the creation of my life.

My body gives me a lot of information about what's happening now, what happened in the past and what's happening in the future.

I use my body as a tool to have more awareness, to have more of me and to perceive everything around me.

When I say something that is not true, i.e., when I lie to myself about what's going on, I get this twisting, heavy sensation between my heart and my solar plexus. When I perceive this feeling in my body, I know I need to ask more questions about what's showing up.

When I choose to be vulnerable with myself and with my body, this is when change can get created. I have to be willing to see what I'm creating in order to be able to make different choices. I have to be willing to be aware of where I'm choosing to limit myself in order to set myself free.

Would you be able to perceive what your body requires if you're not being vulnerable with it?

There is one thing I'd like to impress upon you about all of this: We always have choice. We can choose to have any or all of the elements of intimacy or we can choose not to.

What if you didn't make yourself wrong for either choice?

The key here is to be aware!

Be aware of what your body desires. Be aware of what your being desires. And simply choose what will work in that particular moment. Choice always creates something.

What if you could play in the possibilities of choice?

There is no right or wrong way of doing this. There is simply choice. What would you like to choose today?

WHAT ARE BARRIERS AND BOUNDARIES?

Barriers are the walls we have created throughout our lives to keep ourselves safe from perceived danger. When you put up barriers, you are not only trying to defend against something but you are also cutting off your awareness from everything else around you.

When I was involved in the spiritual community, we referred to these barriers as boundaries. There was great emphasis on knowing your boundaries and expressing them clearly so others don't cross them. They also serve as a way to keep you in check around what to do and not do. Can you perceive the wall in these statements alone?

There is a difference between *knowing you* and *creating barriers*.

When you know what works for you and what doesn't work for you from total space and no judgment, you are able to stay present with that as well as being able to change any of it if you choose. When there is no judgment everything is changeable and fluid.

Barriers and boundaries are so fixed in the rightness and wrongness of everything that they end up becoming so solid it's like a prison you've created for yourself. A prison that confines you and slowly destroys you and your body.

Barriers and boundaries create walls between you, your body and your awareness.

Our bodies are these sensorial organisms. They sense. They feel. We can receive information with our bodies. We can experience the pleasures of this reality with our bodies. When we put up barriers and walls, that makes it a lot more difficult.

Your awareness is your greatest asset!

When you lower your barriers, you are able to perceive and receive energy from everywhere. Perceiving and receiving is not something that we are really taught to have or be in this reality. Personally, I was taught to defend myself and to fight to protect myself.

What if there was something else available?

If you were truly being aware of everything, perceiving all energies and receiving all information, would you have to defend against anything? Would you have to protect yourself from anything or would you just know? Would you be so psychic that all information would be available to you at any time?

Doesn't that sound more fun than hiding behind brick walls?

I had a conversation with Dain once about barriers and boundaries. I asked him what the difference was between the two and he replied:

"It's all bullshit. It's all crap that we use to separate from people, that we use to protect ourselves against something that isn't really truly there. You're an infinite being, would an infinite being really need barriers and boundaries? It's part of the ways that we cut off our awareness, it's part of the ways that we cut off ourselves, not just from receiving from other people, but from receiving from our bodies and gifting to our bodies."

I've noticed, in the destruction of my own barriers, that there are layers. I'll go through one layer of barriers and destroy them. I'll be excited and happy and have a sense of freedom with my body and my being. And then I'll notice another layer, and another layer. I have to keep choosing to lower my barriers and crack open that really tough, hard shell that I have created for myself.

I've also noticed that when I make other people's projections and judgments about me relevant, I create another layer of barriers to protect myself from this awareness. Then I begin to separate myself from people in order to not be aware of what they are thinking about me.

What if none of that was relevant?

What if it didn't matter?

What if it wasn't significant?

As we learned earlier...judgments are really someone else's interesting point of view. They're not real! They're based on their own judgments about themselves and they don't actually have anything to do with me (or you for that matter).

I was at a speaking engagement recently with several other experts in their field. There was a woman that I really wanted to chat with about her business and the possibility of working with her. I tried to chat with her several times and even requested a meeting to talk about working with her.

She never engaged with me and we did not meet. Normally I would have activated the old pattern of "what's wrong with me that she doesn't like me?" Instead, I began asking questions. Later, during her presentation, she spoke of her boss while at a corporate job. She described her as "beautiful with her perfect dress, matching shoes and bag". She went on to describe how this woman had humiliated her in the workplace in front of all her co-workers.

In that moment I knew she had projected her boss on to me. There I was, beautiful, in my pretty dress with my matching shoes and my matching bag. What can I say? I enjoy beauty!

My point is, her not wanting to engage with me had nothing to actually do with me!

Eventually, at another event, we were able to chat and forge a working partnership. This was mostly because I did not make her projection significant and because I did not put up my barriers to her.

When we perceive a judgment and we put up a barrier to it, we are actually choosing to not know what we already know! Those barriers can lock the judgment into your body.

What I've discovered with my body, as well as the clients

I've worked with is that the lockdown ends up creating stiffness, numbness to sensation and numbness to pleasure in the body.

I was working with a client who desired more communion with her body. She had put up so many barriers between herself and her body that she was not able to receive any information from her body.

We worked on "lowering her barriers" and creating space between her and her body. We played with the elements of intimacy between her and her body.

Where was she able to have allowance for her body? When was she allowing herself to trust her body? When could she honor her body? We were even able to find moments of gratitude for her body.

Eventually, as she played with all of this, the communion between her and her body changed. And it kept changing! And growing and expanding. She began having more fun with her body and enjoying all the sensations available.

She even began caring for her body in a completely different way. Longer baths, more time to honor her body, finding ways she could move her body and actually enjoy it.

It was a beautiful journey and such an honor to watch this amazing woman going from lock down to blossoming with joy and ease with her body.

Where are you today with all of this? And if you started making different choices today, where will you be in a year's time? Or 5 year's time?

We all have to start somewhere...and what if where you are today, is totally ok.

PART IV

Your Body & the Elements of Sex

Sex is the body's domain.

If you didn't have a body, would you be able to have sex?

Sex is also one of the most misunderstood areas for ourselves and our bodies in this reality.

I don't know what it was like for you but in my family we were not allowed to talk about sex, much less have it! We could have sex when we got married and then, it became this thing we had *to do* as part of our duties as a wife. Oh brother!

As I mentioned before, when I got caught having sex at the ripe old age of 16, my mother threatened to send me off to Japan. I was promptly grounded for the rest of the year and forbidden to see my boyfriend.

As a Latina, if you had sex you were considered a slut. If you didn't have sex no one wanted to date you. Men are expected to have lots of sex while women are expected to hold out until marriage.

I'm still not clear on how all of that was supposed to work!

In Access Consciousness® we have what are called The Elements of Sex. In this reality, we have actually lumped all of these elements into one big pot of confusing mixed messages.

The distinction between all of the energies involving sex and the body combined with the Elements of Intimacy really gave me a whole new space with my body.

The Elements of Sex are:

1. Copulation
2. Sensuality
3. Sex
4. Sexuality
5. Orgasm
6. Sexualness

COPULATION

Copulation is putting the body parts together. Whichever body parts you prefer...when you put them together you are having copulation. It's what we refer to as having sex in this reality. We'll get to what sex truly is later...

Copulation can be fun and it doesn't necessarily have to mean anything. Some of us are conditioned to believe that if you copulate with someone you must, therefore, get into a relationship with them. I don't know anything about this at all...hehe...

Some say copulation is about bodies playing and having fun together, as if you were playing tennis with someone. Personally, I have experienced this. It is fun. And there are no attachments or commitments to be created. Your body enjoys another person's body and you experience pleasure without the hassle of relationship.

On a different note, copulation does create. The energies between your beings and your bodies creates something. It does not have to be defined or mean anything and you still have to be aware of what you're creating.

If you chose to copulate with a married man or woman, what would that create?

If you chose to copulate with your best friend's boyfriend, what would that create?

If you chose to copulate with someone you picked up at a bar, what would that create?

If you're in a relationship and you chose to copulate with someone else, what would that create?

If you chose to copulate with more that one person at once, what would that create?

Get the picture?

Now, I'm not saying any of these choices are right or wrong. I am simply inviting you to perceive what your choices will create.

Choice creates. Choice creates. Choice creates.

Be aware of what copulation will create and you may save yourself a wee bit of drama in the long run.

I was working with a client years ago. He had come to me about his sexual "issues". He was married and was choosing to visit massage parlors for 'happy endings'.

Over time, we worked on several things. The guilt he was using to hurt himself. The damage he felt he was doing to his wife and marriage. What he was truly searching for when he went for his 'happy' massages. His desire to stop and his "inability" to do so.

We mostly worked on him not making himself wrong for these choices. His wife didn't know and wasn't interested in having sex with him. The massage sessions brought him pleasure and gave him the caring touch he was missing at home. His body enjoyed it. The thing that was causing him the most conflict was the ways in which he was judging himself.

We looked at what this choice was creating for him and it gave him the space to choose something different.

When our work was complete, he thanked me. He had never worked with anyone who held such a space of non-judgment for him.

If there was no judgment, would problems and conflicts exist?

This was also a huge breakthrough for me too. There was a lot of judgment around sex and copulation in my family. I knew I was changing too when this man stepped into my office for facilitation!

This is the miracle of true gifting and receiving.

Sensuality

Sensuality is what the body loves. Being touched, being caressed, being held. Your senses stimulate your body. Your skin, the largest organ in your body receives and perceives sensations.

Imagine if you are completely shut down. Your body is on alert for abuse and your barriers are up.

Are you able to receive? To feel with your body the gentle caress of a lover? The wind stroking your hair? The sun warming your face? The taste of that delicious piece of chocolate fudge cake? The relaxation of a massage?

All of these things can actually nurture and relax your body. Sensuality contributes energy to your body and to your being.

Can you imagine what copulation (sex) would be like if you had **no** sensations with your body?!

For a huge part of my life I was not allowing myself to have sensation and sensuality. It was through my Tantric work, the Access Consciousness® Body Process' and Pole Dancing that I was able to awaken the sensation of my body.

Sensuality is my favorite Element of Sex. Without it, everything is very, very dull.

When I facilitate the Pole Dancing For Consciousness™ classes, there is emphasis on caressing and touching your own body as part of the warm-up we do.

As I do the warm-up, there are so many things that come up for women. Such wrongness around caressing themselves and enjoying their bodies.

Thanks to the tools we are able to change this and I've seen it open women up to their feminine essence.

During one particular class, I was inviting the women to feel the caress of their hair against their skin. One of the women had short hair. She was so open to receiving this that during the warm-up she exclaimed: "I'm gonna let my hair grow out so I can have this!"

A year later, she's grown her hair out and is dressing more sensually and femininely. She is enjoying her body and being a woman!

During another class, a woman surrendered to her body and cried as she said: "I have never been with my body in this way." She later told me that she went home and had the best sex of her life!

How does it get any better than this?!

I've had the pleasure of taking pole dancing classes all over the world. As well as the pleasure of watching many women pole dance. Online and in competitions.

This new trend in using pole dancing to tone your body is pretty cool. And, somewhere along the way, some have lost the art of sensuality. The art of allowing your body to move as she desires. The art of slowing down and enjoying you.

I wonder what it would be like, if every person in the world truly enjoyed their body?

SEX

When Gary Douglas, Co-Founder of Access Consciousness®, talks about sex, he is referring to those times when you are receiving energy.

When you are feeling really good and your body is feeling good and everyone looks at you and flows energy at you. And maybe, sometimes you'd be willing to flow some energy back!

Perceive a time when you were wearing your favorite outfit. And you knew you looked good and felt good and everyone acknowledged you and your energy was expansive and generative.

In Access, sex is referred to as the places where there is a gifting and receiving of energy. You can have sex with everyone in the room. You can have sex outside in nature. You can have sex with the sun or the wind. Remember, sex is *receiving*.

Sometimes, in this reality, the energy of lust is heavily judged. Lust is an energy that the body really enjoys. I know when my body perceives someone lusting after her, she actually moves differently! My butt actually flirts with whoever is lusting after her.

Bodies love to receive this energy. Now, if we could stop

judging men for lusting after us and actually enjoy it...I wonder what that would create?

SEXUALITY

Sexuality is actually a judgment. It is how we define who we will and will not receive energy from in this reality.

For example, if you define yourself as a heterosexual woman and you decide you will only have sex with men, are you going to be able to receive energy from a lesbian woman? A gay man?

When I was in college, I was out dancing with some friends. A beautiful young woman danced her way to me and asked me if I liked girls. I could tell she was flirting with me and, since I didn't consider myself gay, I said "no" and she danced away.

Today, I would be more willing to receive the energy and not cut off whatever her body was willing to gift me. This does not mean I have to copulate with the person but I definitely don't have to cut off my receiving.

Sexuality, as defined in this reality, limits who you can receive from. Bodies gift and receive energy from each other all of the time!

You're an infinite being with a body.

Would an infinite being cut themselves off from receiving anything?

Orgasm

The energy of the creation of your life and the creation of your body.

It's the energy of total presence and awareness with all of the sensations your body has to gift you. The energy of orgasm is the energy of your body and your being really enjoying your life. It's when all the molecules in your body sing with pleasure and joy.

This can be during copulation or it can be just by eating some chocolate!

This reality has defined orgasm as that one moment we all strive for during copulation.

What if your whole life could be an orgasmic experience?

You wouldn't want that for what reason?

There is an energy of creation in orgasmic living. And I don't mean babies!

I mean the joy of living. The joy of having a body.

Did you know money follows joy? If you were truly choosing

the joy of orgasm and the joy of living, there would be no stopping what you could create in your life.

Everything is energy. Does money want to come to a locked-up, shut down pity party or to the party of joy and exuberance?

I was working with a client and she asked me to show her the energy of orgasmic living. While doing a Maestro Symphony body work session on her, we were able to break down the barriers she had created and she ended up having an orgasmic session.

Her body was vibrating and undulating with joy and pleasure. She was laughing loudly and kept screaming "yes, yes yes!". It was truly amazing. It also brought my body pleasure and I also received a healing during the session!

Now, if I could have had this awareness during my session in energy healing school, maybe the tetany I went through could have turned into orgasms rather than a scary experience!

Sexualness

Sexualness is healing, caring, nurturing, joyful, generative, creative, expansive and orgasmic energy. It is an energy you can be with you, with your body and with others.

Sexualness is the space of no judgment.

Sexualness is receiving.

Sexualness is no barriers, total vulnerability.

Notice, there is no mention of copulation here. Sexualness is an energy of being. When you add it to copulation, or to any situation for that matter, the expansiveness that gets created can change the energy of anything.

The true energy of sexualness is almost inconceivable to most people. It was for me too for a long time.

Gary once said: "In order to totally embody sexualness, you have to have the willingness to receive everything and not have a point of view about it."

"In the presence
of total sexualness, nothing
can withstand it's position."
~Dr. Dain Heer

MEN AND SEX

Men think about sex all of the time; they are hard wired to do that. What if that wasn't wrong?

Women are taught that men lusting after you is wrong; that they are perverted or dirty or whatever.

We get ourselves in a double bind, where our bodies like that energy, they are enlivened by that energy, but then it's wrong, it's gross, it's perverted, etc.

What if we could just be present with any energy that is delivered?

What if we didn't judge energy?

Energy is just energy. It is neither right nor wrong.

What if we didn't make men wrong for anything?

What invitation can we be, as women, to allow men to be men?

What if we didn't choose to separate men and women?

HAVING A HEALING BODY

This is definitely not something we are taught in this reality and yet I have found it's one of the most important awarenesses we can acknowledge about ourselves.

Our bodies, as creators of consciousness have healing abilities.

Here's an article I wrote about a particularly life transforming event. It was the first time I acknowledged my body's healing capacities.

It was also the first time I had experienced a simultaneous healing with a man who also had a healing body.

As you read this article, I ask you to ponder...if there had been any judgment in either of our worlds, would this have been created?

Does your body have abilities you haven't acknowledged?

Did you know bodies have healing abilities that can facilitate and contribute consciousness and awareness?

This isn't exactly something we are taught in school, is it? Developing Pole Dancing For Consciousness™ has created a space for me to dive deeper into the possibilities with bodies in a way that I never expected.

As much as I know in this moment, what happened at an Access Consciousness 7 Day event in Costa Rica facilitated me into even more awareness of my body's capacities.

I'd love to tell you what occurred....

We were at the pool one night and I was asked to dance for everyone. I said no at first. Then, I noticed that the energy for a dance was light and expansive so I said yes.

I picked a song, put on a shirt and stood there tuning into the energy of what was required in that moment.

The music began to permeate the molecules of my body. Letting go of the mind, allowing my body to lead, I danced by the side of the pool under the moonlight.

It was so nurturing and delicious for my body. Seduced by the night air, the water, the music, the energy and the people around me, I found myself slipping seductively into the pool touching and caressing those who were willing to receive.

As I made my way around the pool I could hear someone talking. My body instantly made the demand of total attention. I walked towards him and said, "Are you still talking?"

As I got close to him I slowly peeled off my shirt. My arm reached around him and my hand touched his back. My body pressed against him and our eyes locked orgasmically, aggressively, present with each other.

Even though my feet could not touch the pool floor, I

somehow lead us around the pool. We were conquered to the energy that had been created...Quiet, intense, sexy and indescribable by words alone.

I became aware that everyone had their eyes on us. My body pushed him away and I smiled. Everyone shouted, clapped and laughed.

Shocked and in awe, this beautiful man began to shake and release tears from his body. I gave him some space to be with what was showing up.

Women attempted to comfort him but he did not want to be touched. Eventually, I moved towards him and asked him to look at me. He wouldn't.

I held him from behind and put my hand over his heart. He allowed me to do this. He still couldn't speak to what had just occurred.

I could barely get a sense of what had been created. I was acutely aware of the judgments around me and the shifting of energy. I chose to give him more space and create some space for myself as well.

I made my way to the bar to sit. I lowered my barriers and became present to the energy around me.

Eventually, he joined me and told me what he could about what had transpired. He said he'd never experienced that kind presence and kindness with a woman.

He stated that my body and I were an invitation for him to have more consciousness and that he is forever changed. I wondered what he would demand from the women in his life now...I wondered what contribution that would be to him, to everyone around him and to the world.

We facilitate each other and I get that this beautiful, sexy man has received what I knew was possible between a man and a woman. Something occurred that is beyond this reality.

I am also forever changed, as I have never experienced this kind of presence with a man before. I am filled with gratitude for his contribution to my world.

Over the next few days, he proceeded to show me a reality with men I thought I would never be able to have.

He is kind, generous, honoring, funny, smart and a gentleman who is steadfast in his choices. I watch him begin to make choices for himself that will create a different reality for him and those around him.

Our bodies facilitated a healing in that moment that is still unfolding in my Universe. I am curious about what else will show up for me.

I am so grateful that our bodies were able to receive each other in this way. What else is possible now that I have never imagined?

What would it take for me to continue discovering the endless possibilities of what is being created?

Do you have a healing body?

A body that can heal just by your very presence?

What if you acknowledged this for yourself?

What would your life be like if you chose to embrace your body's abilities?

PART V

PRACTICAL TOOLS FOR PRAGMATIC CHANGE

In the following section I'd like to invite you to put into practice some of what we've looked at throughout this book.

Are you ready to commit to more communion with your body?

Are you ready to allow your body's wisdom to contribute to the creation of your life?

Are you ready to awaken, embody and unleash the magnificent you into the world?

Getting out of lockdown with your body must include your body in that process.

I've detailed some of my favorite home play exercises. These are the tools I continue to use to this day to keep opening myself up, to destroy the barriers I've created and have the orgasmic life and living I know is possible.

Would you be willing to turn on every molecule in your body?

Shall we play?

NOT SURE IF YOU HAVE BARRIERS?

Being able to let go of your barriers begins with being aware of when you are choosing them.

This home play exercise is designed to give you a sense of what barriers may feel like in your body.

1. Lay down somewhere comfortable and take a few deep breaths. Connect with your body. Breathe.

2. Expand your energy out into the Universe. As far as you can. Fill the room with your being and invite your body to do the same.

3. Now, do your best to tighten every single muscle in your body. Squinch your toes, squeeze your buttocks and your genitals, clench your fists, your shoulders and your face

4. Hold for 5 seconds.

5. Now relax. Relax everything. Inhale and exhale. Breathe. Expand your energy out again.

6. Repeat steps 1-4 several times until you get the sense of when you are contracting and when you're expanding.

When I first did this exercise I could not even perceive what relaxing my body meant. I had to do it several times over several days to get the sense of relaxing and contracting.

This exercise facilitated me into really getting that sense of when I was locking up my body (contracting), when my barriers were going up and when I was shutting down.

Once you have a visceral sense of contraction, you can be more aware of when you're choosing to put up your barriers. The senses your body is giving you is part of having that awareness.

Your body can give you information of the places where you are holding tension in your body and the places where you are able to relax.

Go to:

YourBodyIsConsciousneness.com/secretbonuses

To gain access to a guided meditation that includes this powerful tool!

LOWERING YOUR BARRIERS

The cool thing about barriers is that we have created them, so we can choose to let them go and lower them. This can be as easy as asking them...

With the above exercise and your new found awareness of when you're choosing barriers, you can now simply say:

"Lower my barriers"

"Lower my barriers"

"Lower my barriers"

In some situation you may actually need to push them down...energetically of course!

As you lower your barriers, simultaneously expand your energy out. Here are a few simple steps to practice this as well:

1. Find a comfortable place to sit and feel your butt on the chair

2. Perceive and be present with your body. Feels your toes, your legs, your belly, your chest, your head

3. Breathe in to your belly and allow it to expand out.

4. As you exhale, allowing your belly to come towards

your spine. And as you do this, expand your energy out; expand your body out; occupying the entire space of the room that you are in and further.

5. Now, think of someone you're having an issue with. Allow them to come into your awareness and notice what happens in your body.

Did your barriers pop up?

6. Now, lower your barriers, push them down if you need to...more, more, more...expand out....lower your barriers...

Did that shift anything for you?

We can most certainly let go of all of our barriers and be the vulnerability that is required for lasting change and true happiness.

It may just take a little bit of practice.

Are you willing to be patient with yourself as you embark on this new adventure?

There's another guided meditation including this home play exercise here:

YourBodyIsConsciousneness.com/secretbonuses

Sign up for your secret bonuses today!

Shaking It All Out!

This is the best Tantric/QiGong exercise for getting out of lockdown I have ever experienced and taught. It literally breaks down the locked up patterns that are held in your body.

I would suggest you do this exercise every other day. Starting with 3 minutes on the first day and adding a minute every time you do it.

Start slow and build. You want to be aware of your body as you do this.

If it does not feel good, don't do it!

Stay present with your neck and your knees.

1. Download *Communiqué: Approach Spiral* by Michael Shrieve from your favorite music store. I have found this to be the most effective song for this exercise.

2. Set a time for the amount of time you'll be doing this exercise

3. Stand with your feet planted firmly on the ground

4. Slightly bend your knees

5. As the music begins, start bouncing. Gently at first

until you get the hang of it. As the music progresses bounce a bit more...as I mentioned, build up to this

6. Keep your feet planted on the ground – maintaining connection with the Earth

7. The target is to get everything moving! Your genitals, your shoulders, your arms, your buttocks. Everything shaking and bouncing!

8. When the timer goes off, slow down gently. Please DO NOT just stop. Slow down until you come to a complete standstill

9. Stay present with your body, notice the energy moving.

10. Lay down and rest the same amount of time that you did the exercise. Stay present with your body. Allow your body to move as it requires.

Eventually you want to be able to shake for the entirety of the song.

As your body unlocks, you may have a release of sorts. Laughing, crying, the sensation of being expanded may all occur! What else is possible?!

What would it take to have fun with all of these??

I've included a video of this tool in your Secret Bonuses page. Have you signed up yet?

YourBodyIsConsciousneness.com/SecretBonuses

ALLOWING YOUR BODY TO MOVE

I am a dancing enthusiast so you knew this one had to be coming...

It's a fun home play designed to invite you to let go and allow your body to move...the way he or she desires to move!

1. Choose your favorite song

2. Close your eyes and breathe it in

3. Get really present with your body and don't move... until your body wants to move

4. Get out of the way and allow your body to move...no matter what it looks like.

5. You can ask "Body, how would you like to move to this song?" And see what shows up.

6. Do this with several different kinds of songs, even songs YOU don't think you'd like...allow your body to choose the song!

Even if you stand there the whole time not moving and perceiving your body that is ok.

What would it take for you to not judge you during this home play?

Sometimes I hear a song on the radio and I'm driving around and I'm super excited about the song. And I think: "I'm *so* going to dance to this song in my next class!" And when I play the song in class and really tune into my body, turns out my body doesn't like it at all!

What if you could play with this and see what shows up? Would you be willing to be silly? To have fun with your body?

Simply notice what gets created with your body?

For fun, here are some of my favorite songs to move to:

Ginuwine	Pony
AWOLNATION	Sail
Kings of Leon	Closer
Katy Perry	Dark Horse
Eminem	Shake That Ass For Me (feat. Nate Dogg)
Sam Smith	Lay Me Down (Acoustic)
Michael Jackson	Dirty Diana
Apocalyptica	Nothing Else Matters
Joe Cocker	Leave Your Hat On
The Hit Crew	You Sexy Thing
La Mazz	When Doves Cry
Flo Rida	Right Round
The Hot Damns	Wicked Games

Getting to Know the Language of Your Body

Asking your body questions is a great way to get to know the language of your body.

Every body is different. What is yummy for you may not be yummy for others!

It is also a great way to invite the consciousness of your body into contributing to the creation of your life.

Earlier we looked at *Following the Energy.* Let's recap this a bit as you will be asking questions and following the energy to what will create more.

First, you ask your body a question. Then, tunc in to the energy and choose by following the energy.

If the energy is *light and expansive*, then this is true for you.

If the energy is *heavy and contracts*, then this is a lie for you.

Follow the lightness. Follow what is true for you.

You can use this tool to begin choosing what works for your body.

We sometimes override what our bodies desire in favor of

what we desire. And, at other times, what is light for our bodies does not make any sense to us!

What if, for just one day, you used this tool and chose only what was light for your body? I wonder what awareness you would gain on that day?

If you didn't have a body, would you need clothes? Food? A car? Hugs?

The joy of having a body is about enJOYing your body. And everything we have on this beautiful planet is for your body.

Enjoying your body can begin with simply allowing your body to choose what he/she would like.

You can start playing with this right away by being in the question about anything and everything having to do with your body.

Here's a list of questions to play with everyday.

Body, what would you like to wear today?

Body, what would you like to eat today?

Body, what would you like to do for fun today?

Body, what is healing for you?

Body, what is caring for you?

Body, what would it be like to be vulnerable with you?

Body, what would it be like to have honor for you?

Body, what would it be like to trust you?

Simply ask the questions and allow your body to give you the energy of what it would like.

You can play with one at a time or play with all of them!

GRATITUDE FOR YOUR BODY

Would you be willing, just for today, to find 5 things to be grateful for with your body?

Some suggestions may be...

Did you wake up today?

What is healthy with your body?

Did you enjoy your food today?

Go for a walk and notice everything your body is also aware of. The birds singing. The sun shining. The snow falling. Whatever is happening for you today.

Would you be willing to be grateful for everything you are gifting and receiving with the Earth?

A Sweet Farewell...For Now

This book had been asking to be written for a while now. Between life, love and creation, I hadn't made the time to sit down and just write.

In July of 2016, I took myself and my body to a remote Air BnB in the Cayman Islands for two weeks.

Receiving the nurturing care of the ocean, the wind, the sun and the sand, I wrote my first draft in 5 days.

Everyday I asked questions. I asked my body for contribution and awareness on what to write next.

What did my body desire to contribute to you?

Your Body as the Creation of Consciousness was completed in less than two weeks and launched into the world within a month.

What if you allowed your body to contribute to you in this way?

What if you didn't judge your creations?

What if it was easier than you could possibly imagine?

You may want to read this a few times...there's a lot of juicy nuggets to invite you into this possibility and beyond...

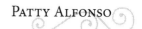

How does it get any better than that?™

What else is possible now?®

SECRET BONUSES JUST FOR YOU!

Have you signed up for the *Secret Bonuses Membership* page? I have so many more things to gift you on this site!

To access the site for free go to:

YourBodyIsConsciousneness.com/secretbonuses

and enter your email address.

I've created a place with additional resources, inspirational videos and quotes, some samples of what Pole Dancing For Consciousness looks like, meditation and receiving excrcises and much more!

When you join my list, you'll also receive articles, video content and special invitations to all of my upcoming webinars, classes and exclusive live events.

These resources will guide you in having more joy, sensation, pleasure and fun in your life.

What if the purpose of life is to have fun?!

Enjoy these gifts. Thank you again for purchasing my book! It's been an honor to share my life with you!

I hope to see you, someday, around the globe!

ABOUT THE AUTHOR

A catalyst for transformation, Patty Alfonso is an internationally acclaimed speaker, facilitator and author. She is a world traveler with a global business that inspires her clients to create magic in their life with their business, their bodies and in their relationships.

Patty is the creator of Pole Dancing for Consciousness™ and The Essence of You™. Her kind, witty and sharp facilitation invites participants into having more ease, joy, pleasure and communion.

Born and raised in Guaynabo, Puerto Rico, Patty received her Bachelor's Degree in Sociology from Emory University. She is certified as a Body/Mind Counselor and Energy Healing Therapist. Patty's desire to continue growing and empower her clients, led her to Access Consciousness®, where she is a Certified Facilitator.

For more information about Patty's work, go to:
www.PattyAlfonso.Sexy

ALL OF LIFE COMES TO ME WITH EASE, JOY AND GLORY®!

Made in the USA
Middletown, DE
28 September 2018